Diabetic Diet
Cookbook for Beginners
2024

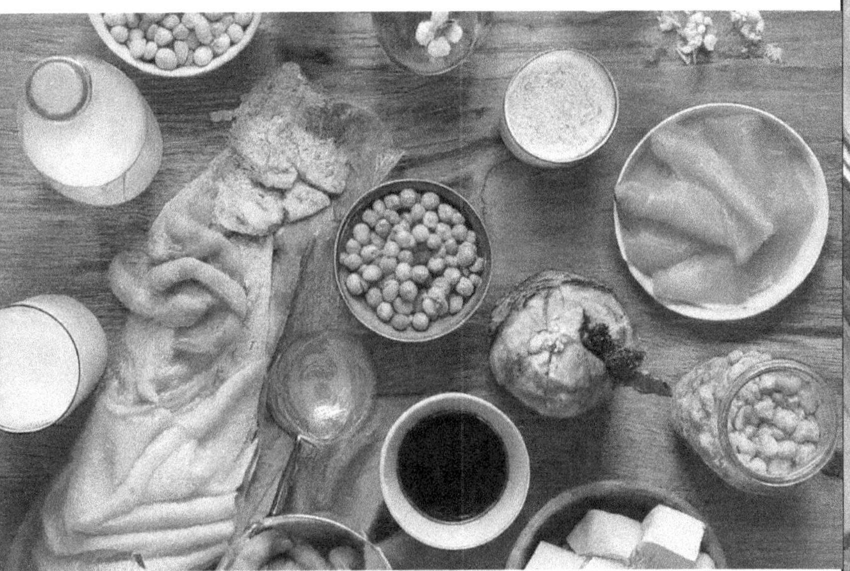

2000 Days of Easy, Healthy & Delicious Recipes:
Low-Carb, Low-Sugar, High-Fiber Meals for Type 1, Type 2, Gestational Diabetes & Prediabetes

Avery Stoneheart

Table of Contents

Introduction 3

Chapter 1: Mastering the Menu 6

   Demystifying Diabetes and Delicious Eats 6

Chapter 2: Building Your Healthy Haven 9

   Essential Staples for the Diabetic Kitchen 9

Chapter 3: Recipes for Breakfast 12

Chapter 4: Recipes for Lunch 29

Chapter 5: Recipes for Dinner 52

Chapter 6: Creative Snacks and Sides 75

Chapter 7: Desserts and Special Occasions 93

   Diabetic-Friendly Holiday Cheer: Tips from a Registered Dietitian .. 104

   BONUS CHAPTER 107

   DIABETES MEAL PLAN TRACKER 107

   DIABETES DIET MONTHLY TRACKER 108

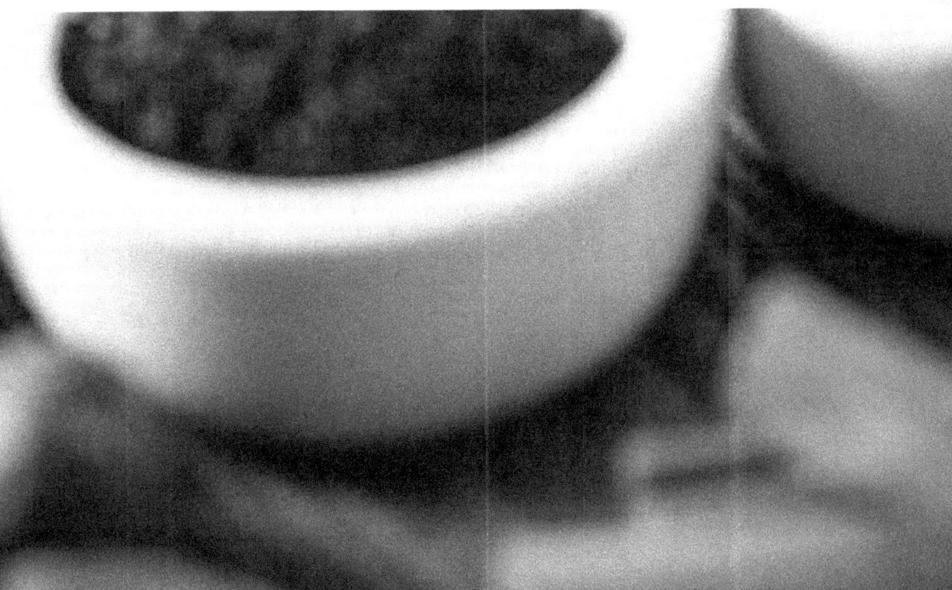

Introduction

Welcome to Your Personalized Plate: A Delicious Path to Diabetes Management

Hey there! I'm Avery Stoneheart, your friendly neighborhood registered dietitian and certified diabetes educator. For over 20 years, I've witnessed firsthand the struggles and triumphs of individuals navigating life with diabetes. I understand the frustration of confusing dietary guidelines, the constant battle against cravings, and the longing for a vibrant life beyond restrictions.

But here's the secret I've learned: ***diabetes doesn't have to dictate your culinary adventures.*** In fact, with the right knowledge and a dash of creativity, you can unlock a world of flavor-packed meals that nourish your body and empower you to live life on your terms.

That's why I'm thrilled to introduce you to ***"Your Personalized Plate: A Delicious Path to Diabetes Management."*** Forget bland, one-size-fits-all recipes and complicated calculations. This isn't just a cookbook; it's your personal guide to reclaiming your culinary freedom, packed with over 2000 days' worth of mouthwatering recipes tailored specifically to your needs.

What makes this book different?

1. **Personalized for You:** Whether you're managing Type 1, Type 2, Gestational Diabetes, or Prediabetes, you'll find recipes designed to support your unique health goals.
2. **Flavorful and Functional:** Forget the sacrifice! We've created delicious dishes that are low-carb, low-calorie, high-fiber, low-sugar, and heart-healthy, all without compromising taste.
3. **Beginner-Friendly:** No culinary expertise required! Clear instructions, readily available ingredients, and helpful tips ensure you can whip up delicious meals with confidence, even if you're new to the kitchen.

But it's not just about the recipes. This book is your ultimate companion on your journey to well-being. You'll find:

- **Science Made Simple:** I'll break down the science of diabetes management into bite-sized, easy-to-understand explanations, empowering you to make informed choices about your food.
- **Expert Hacks and Tips:** From smart substitutions to meal planning strategies, I'll share my years of experience to help you navigate everyday challenges and celebrate special occasions without sacrificing your health.
- **Real-Life Inspiration:** Get motivated by heartwarming stories from individuals who have transformed their lives through delicious, diabetes-friendly eating.

Are you ready to:

1. Ditch the deprivation and embrace a world of vibrant flavors?
2. Feel energized and empowered to manage your diabetes with confidence?
3. Discover a world of delicious possibilities that nourish your body and soul?

Then turn the page and embark on a delicious journey to a healthier, happier you!

Remember, you're not alone in this. Let's create a future where food fuels your passion for life, not limitations.

See you inside!
Warmly,
Avery Stoneheart, RD, CDE

Chapter 1: Mastering the Menu

Demystifying Diabetes and Delicious Eats

Hold onto your forks, food explorers! Before we unleash our inner chefs with diabetes-friendly recipes, let's crack the code on how your body interacts with food. Think of this chapter as your personalized decoder ring, unlocking the secrets to mastering your health through delicious meals.

The Diabetes Detectives:

First up, let's meet the different diabetes suspects:

1. **Type 1:** Picture this – your body's the bouncer, and insulin's the VIP pass for sugar to enter your cells. In Type 1, the bouncer's gone MIA, leaving sugar stranded outside, causing chaos.

2. **Type 2:** Here, the bouncer exists, but he's gotten a bit drowsy. He lets some sugar in, but not always efficiently, leading to similar disruptions.

3. **Gestational:** This temporary guest shows up during pregnancy, temporarily messing with how your body handles sugar.

4. **Prediabetes:** Imagine a warning sign – your blood sugar's higher than normal, but not quite high enough for a formal diagnosis.

Food, the Flavorful Maestro:

Now, let's talk about the conductor orchestrating your blood sugar symphony – food! What you choose to eat plays a starring role, so understanding their individual melodies is key.

1. **Carbohydrates:** These are the energetic performers, but some, like refined sugars and white bread, belt out loud, spiking your blood sugar. Others, like whole grains and vegetables, have soothing harmonies, releasing energy gradually.
2. **Fiber:** Imagine your digestive BFF, harmonizing with carbohydrates to slow down their sugar release and keep you feeling full for longer.
3. **Sugar:** This tempting siren can lead to blood sugar mayhem. While some natural sugars in fruits are okay, added sugars are best kept offstage.
4. **Proteins and Fats:** These are the supporting actors, providing essential nutrients and keeping you satisfied, preventing you from reaching for sugary snacks mid-performance.

Glycemic Index and Load:

Ever ridden a roller coaster? That's kind of how different foods affect your blood sugar. The Glycemic Index (GI) tells you how quickly a food raises your sugar levels, while the Glycemic Load (GL) considers the quantity and type of carbohydrate. By understanding these, you can choose foods that create a smooth, gentle ride for your blood sugar.

Label Language:

Food labels are your backstage passes, revealing the ingredients behind each dish. Learn to decipher the carbohydrate content, fiber, and added sugars to make informed choices. Remember, "serving size" is the spotlight – don't get fooled by hidden sugars lurking in seemingly healthy options!

Chapter 2: Building Your Healthy Haven

Essential Staples for the Diabetic Kitchen

Welcome back, food adventurers! Now that we've demystified the science behind diabetes and food, let's transform your kitchen into a haven of delicious, health-promoting ingredients. Think of this chapter as your shopping list and pantry makeover guide, packed with tips and tricks to equip you for culinary success.

Non-Perishable Pantry Powerhouses:

1. **Grains:** Opt for whole-wheat options like brown rice, quinoa, oats, and whole-wheat pasta for sustained energy and fiber.

2. **Beans and Lentils:** These protein and fiber powerhouses add variety and heartiness to meals. Stock up on canned or dried varieties for versatility.

3. **Nuts and Seeds:** Packed with healthy fats, protein, and fiber, these are perfect for snacking, adding to salads, or incorporating into dishes. Choose unsalted and raw varieties for better control.

4. **Spices and Herbs:** Elevate the flavor of your food without added sugar or sodium. Stock up on essentials like garlic powder, cumin, chili powder, oregano, and basil.

5. **Dried Fruits and Unsweetened Nuts:** Satisfy your sweet tooth naturally with dried fruits like cranberries, raisins, and unsweetened nut butters. Opt for smaller portions to manage sugar intake.

6. **Canned Vegetables:** No time for fresh? Opt for low-sodium canned vegetables like black beans, diced tomatoes, and corn for quick and convenient meal additions.
7. **Healthy Oils:** Olive oil, avocado oil, and canola oil are great for cooking and salad dressings. Opt for extra virgin options for higher quality and flavor.
8. **Vinegars:** Add a zing to your dishes with balsamic vinegar, apple cider vinegar, and red wine vinegar. Experiment with different flavors to create unique dressings and marinades.

Fresh Fridge Friends:

1. **Leafy Greens:** Spinach, kale, romaine lettuce, and collard greens are packed with vitamins, minerals, and fiber. Keep them washed and ready for salads, wraps, or smoothies.
2. **Colorful Vegetables:** Bell peppers, broccoli, carrots, cauliflower, and zucchini add vibrant colors and essential nutrients to your diet. Roast, stir-fry, or enjoy them raw with dips.
3. **Fruits:** Berries, apples, pears, and citrus fruits are excellent sources of vitamins, fiber, and antioxidants. Enjoy them whole, sliced, or blended into smoothies.
4. **Lean Protein Sources:** Skinless chicken breasts, lean ground turkey, fish, and tofu provide essential protein without excess saturated fat.
5. **Eggs:** A versatile and affordable protein source, perfect for breakfast, lunch, or dinner. Opt for omega-3 enriched eggs for added benefits.
6. **Low-Fat Dairy Products:** Unsweetened yogurt, skim milk, and low-fat cheeses offer calcium and protein without excess fat.

Stocking Smarts:

1. **Plan your meals:** Knowing what you'll cook helps you buy what you need and avoid impulse purchases.
2. **Read food labels:** Pay attention to serving sizes, carbohydrate content, and added sugars.
3. **Shop in bulk:** Buy staples like grains, nuts, and spices in bulk to save money and reduce packaging waste.
4. **Don't forget frozen:** Frozen fruits and vegetables are flash-frozen at peak ripeness, preserving nutrients and offering convenience.
5. **Fight food waste:** Store fruits and vegetables properly, utilize leftovers creatively, and freeze portions for later use.

Sweet Swaps and Savory Subs:

1. **Craving sweets?** Instead of sugary desserts, try Greek yogurt with berries, baked apples with cinnamon, or dark chocolate with nuts.
2. **Pasta craving?** Opt for whole-wheat pasta or spiralized vegetables like zucchini noodles.
3. **Need bread?** Choose whole-wheat bread or make your own using healthy flours like almond flour or coconut flour.
4. **Rice is out?** Try quinoa, barley, or cauliflower rice for lower carb alternatives.
5. **Sweetener dilemma?** Use stevia, erythritol, or monk fruit extract in moderation for sweetness without the sugar spike.

Remember, building a healthy pantry is a journey, not a destination. Experiment, have fun, and remember, small changes can make a big difference in your health and well-being. Happy shopping and cooking!

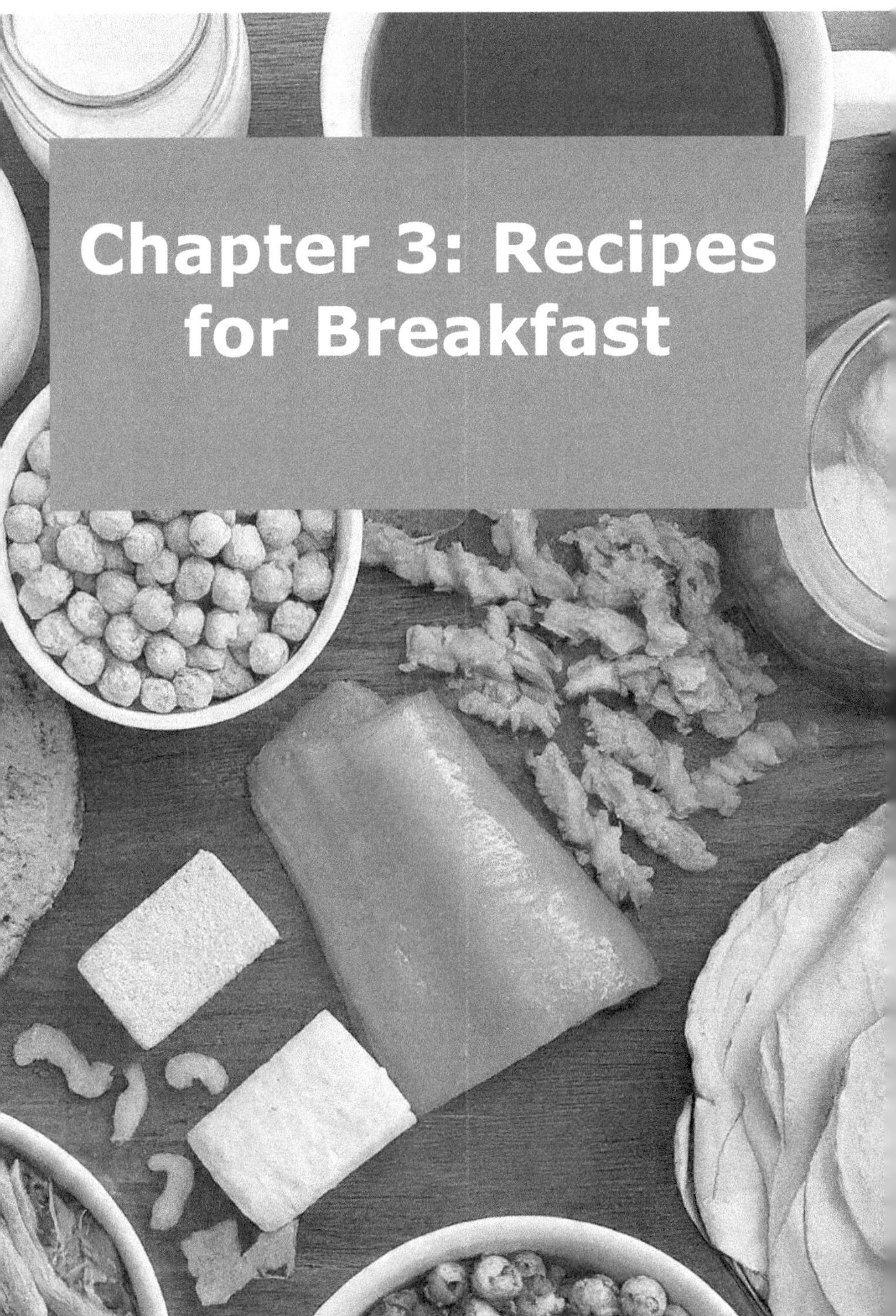

Chapter 3: Recipes for Breakfast

Diabetic-Friendly Recipe Guide:

Savory Mushroom & Lentil Scramble (Vegetarian):

Ingredients:

- 1 tbsp olive oil
- 1 cup chopped mushrooms (cremini, shiitake, or your choice)
- 1/2 bell pepper, chopped
- 1/4 onion, chopped
- 1 cup cooked brown lentils
- 1 cup chopped spinach
- 1/2 tsp turmeric
- 1/2 tsp cumin
- 1/4 tsp chili powder
- 2 eggs
- 2 tbsp unsweetened almond milk
- 1 whole-wheat tortilla (optional)
- 1/2 avocado, sliced (optional)

Instructions:

1. Heat olive oil in a pan over medium heat. Add mushrooms, bell pepper, and onion. Sauté until softened, about 5 minutes.
2. Add lentils, spinach, turmeric, cumin, and chili powder. Stir to combine and cook for 2 minutes.
3. In a separate bowl, whisk eggs with almond milk. Pour into the pan with the veggies and lentils.
4. Scramble the eggs gently until cooked through, about 3-4 minutes.

5. Serve on a whole-wheat tortilla or with avocado slices, enjoying every bite without impacting your blood sugar significantly.

Nutritional Information:

- Calories: 350
- Carbohydrates: 25g
- Fiber: 7g
- Protein: 20g
- Fat: 15g

Tips:

- Use low-sodium vegetable broth instead of almond milk for extra savory flavor.
- Add additional vegetables like chopped zucchini or asparagus for more variety.
- Substitute the eggs with 1/4 cup of crumbled tofu for a vegan option.

2. Beetroot & Goat Cheese Smoothie with Berries (Vegan):

Ingredients:

- 1 medium beet, cooked and chopped
- 1 cup unsweetened almond milk
- 1/2 cup frozen berries (mixed, blueberry, or your choice)
- 1 cup spinach
- 1/4 tsp stevia (optional)
- 1 tbsp dollop of goat cheese (optional)
- 1/4 cup granola
- 1/4 cup chopped nuts (almonds, walnuts, or your choice)

Instructions:

1. Blend together beet, almond milk, berries, and spinach until smooth.
2. Taste and add stevia for sweetness, if desired.
3. Pour into a glass and top with goat cheese (optional), granola, and chopped nuts for added protein and crunch.

Nutritional Information:

- Calories: 250
- Carbohydrates: 30g
- Fiber: 6g
- Protein: 8g
- Fat: 10g

Tips:

- Use cooked beets from the grocery store to save time.
- Substitute the goat cheese with 1/4 cup of plain Greek yogurt for a lower-fat option.
- Add a scoop of unflavored protein powder for a more filling smoothie.

3. Salmon & Veggie Frittata with Arugula Salad:

Ingredients:

- 4 eggs
- 1/4 cup chopped fresh herbs (dill, parsley, or your choice)
- 1/4 tsp salt
- 1/4 tsp black pepper
- 1 cup chopped spinach
- 1/2 cup chopped asparagus
- 1/4 cup cherry tomatoes, halved
- 1/2 cup cooked and flaked salmon (canned or baked)
- 1 cup arugula salad
- Balsamic vinaigrette dressing

Instructions:

1. Preheat oven to 375°F (190°C). Grease a 9-inch pie dish.
2. In a bowl, whisk eggs with herbs, salt, and pepper.
3. Layer spinach, asparagus, and cherry tomatoes in the prepared dish.
4. Top with flaked salmon and pour in the egg mixture.
5. Bake for 25-30 minutes, or until the eggs are set and the frittata is golden brown.
6. Serve warm with a side of arugula salad drizzled with balsamic vinaigrette.

Nutritional Information:

- Calories: 350
- Carbohydrates: 15g
- Fiber: 2g
- Protein: 30g
- Fat: 20g

Tips:

- Use low-fat or fat-free cheese for a lower-fat option.
- Substitute the salmon with lean chicken breast or tofu for a different protein source.
- Add other vegetables like sliced bell peppers or zucchini for more variety.

4. Mushroom & Swiss Omelet with Whole-wheat Toast:

Ingredients:

- 1 tbsp olive oil
- 1 cup chopped mushrooms
- 1/4 onion, chopped
- 1 cup shredded Swiss cheese (reduced-fat)
- 2 eggs
- 1 whole-wheat toast slice
- 1/2 tomato, sliced (optional)
- 1/4 avocado, sliced (optional)

Instructions:

1. Heat olive oil in a pan over medium heat. Add mushrooms and onion. Sauté until softened, about 5 minutes.
2. In a separate bowl, whisk eggs with a pinch of salt and pepper.
3. Stir half of the shredded cheese into the egg mixture.
4. Pour the egg mixture into the pan with the mushrooms and onions.
5. Tilt the pan to spread the eggs evenly.
6. Once the bottom starts to set, sprinkle remaining cheese on one half of the omelet.
7. Fold the other half over the cheese and cook for another minute or two, until the cheese melts and the eggs are cooked through.
8. Serve the omelet on a whole-wheat toast slice with sliced tomato and avocado (optional).

Nutritional Information:

- Calories: 300
- Carbohydrates: 20g
- Fiber: 2g
- Protein: 20g
- Fat: 15g

Tips:

- Use low-fat Swiss cheese to reduce saturated fat content.
- Add chopped spinach or other vegetables to the omelet for added nutrients.
- Substitute the eggs with 1/4 cup of crumbled tofu for a vegan option.

5. Breakfast Bowl with Black Beans, Avocado, and Salsa:

Ingredients:

- 1/2 cup cooked black beans (low-sodium)
- 1/2 avocado, sliced
- 1/4 cup salsa (low-sugar)
- 2 scrambled eggs
- 1/4 cup cherry tomatoes, halved
- 1/4 cup chopped cilantro
- 1 tbsp lime juice
- 1 whole-wheat tortilla (optional)

Instructions:

1. Layer black beans, avocado, and salsa in a bowl.
2. Top with scrambled eggs, cherry tomatoes, and cilantro.
3. Drizzle with lime juice and serve with a whole-wheat tortilla (optional).

Nutritional Information:

- Calories: 300
- Carbohydrates: 30g
- Fiber: 8g
- Protein: 15g
- Fat: 10g

Tips:

- Use canned black beans rinsed and drained for convenience.
- Choose a low-sugar salsa to manage carbohydrate intake.
- Substitute the eggs with 1/4 cup of cooked quinoa for a plant-based protein option.

7. Greek Yogurt Parfait with Berries and Chia Seeds:

Ingredients:

- 1 cup plain Greek yogurt (low-fat or non-fat)
- 1/2 cup unsweetened berries (mixed, blueberry, or your choice)
- 2 tbsp chia seeds
- 1/4 tsp stevia (optional)
- 1/4 cup chopped nuts (almonds, walnuts, or your choice)
- 1/4 tsp ground cinnamon (optional)

Instructions:

1. Layer yogurt, berries, and chia seeds in a parfait glass or container.
2. Sweeten with stevia, if desired.
3. Top with chopped nuts and sprinkle with cinnamon for added flavor and crunch.

Nutritional Information:

- Calories: 250
- Carbohydrates: 20g
- Fiber: 5g
- Protein: 20g
- Fat: 5g

Tips:

- Use unsweetened fruit instead of berries for a lower-sugar option.
- Substitute chia seeds with flaxseeds for similar benefits.
- Add a scoop of unflavored protein powder for an extra protein boost.

8. Mushroom & Spinach Quesadilla with Black Beans:

Ingredients:

- 1 tbsp olive oil
- 1 cup chopped mushrooms
- 1 cup chopped spinach
- 1/2 tsp chili powder
- 1/4 tsp cumin
- 1/2 cup mashed black beans (low-sodium)
- 1 whole-wheat tortilla
- 1/4 cup shredded cheese (low-fat mozzarella or another variety)

Instructions:

1. Heat olive oil in a pan over medium heat. Add mushrooms and cook until softened, about 5 minutes.
2. Add spinach and cook until wilted.
3. Stir in chili powder and cumin.
4. Spread mashed black beans on one half of the tortilla.
5. Top with the mushroom and spinach mixture and sprinkle with cheese.
6. Fold the tortilla in half and cook on a pan or grill until golden brown and cheese melts.

Nutritional Information:

- Calories: 300
- Carbohydrates: 30g
- Fiber: 7g
- Protein: 15g
- Fat: 10g

Tips:

- Use low-fat cheese to reduce saturated fat content.
- Add other vegetables like chopped bell peppers or onions for more variety.
- Use two small whole-wheat tortillas instead of one large one for better portion control.

9. Rhubarb & Strawberry Smoothie with Protein Powder:

Ingredients:

- 1 cup unsweetened almond milk
- 1/2 cup frozen strawberries
- 1/2 cup chopped rhubarb
- 1 cup spinach
- 1 scoop unflavored protein powder
- 1/4 cup granola (low-sugar)
- 1/4 cup chopped nuts (optional)

Instructions:

1. Blend almond milk, strawberries, rhubarb, spinach, and protein powder until smooth.
2. Pour into a glass and top with granola and chopped nuts (optional).

Nutritional Information:

- Calories: 300
- Carbohydrates: 35g
- Fiber: 7g
- Protein: 25g
- Fat: 10g

Tips:

- Use fresh or frozen rhubarb, depending on season and availability.
- Sweeten with stevia or a small amount of natural sweetener if desired.
- Substitute the protein powder with 1/4 cup of plain Greek yogurt for a thicker smoothie.

10. Turkey Sausage & Veggie Scramble with Whole-grain Toast:

Ingredients:

- 1 tbsp olive oil
- 1/2 cup cooked turkey sausage (low-fat)
- 1/2 bell pepper, chopped
- 1/4 onion, chopped
- 1 cup chopped mushrooms
- 1 cup chopped spinach
- 2 eggs
- 1/4 tsp paprika
- 1/4 tsp garlic powder
- 1/4 tsp onion powder
- 1 slice whole-grain toast
- 1/2 tomato, sliced (optional)
- 1/4 avocado, sliced (optional)

Instructions:

1. Heat olive oil in a pan over medium heat. Add turkey sausage, bell pepper, and onion. Cook until sausage is browned and vegetables are softened.
2. Add mushrooms and spinach. Cook until spinach wilts.
3. Scramble eggs in a separate bowl.
4. Add eggs to the pan with the vegetables and cook until scrambled through.
5. Season with paprika, garlic powder, and onion powder.
6. Serve the scramble on a slice of whole-grain toast with sliced tomato and avocado (optional).

Nutritional Information:

- Calories: 350
- Carbohydrates: 25g
- Fiber: 3g
- Protein: 30g
- Fat: 15g

Tips:

- Use turkey sausage links or ground turkey, depending on preference.
- Add other vegetables like chopped zucchini or broccoli for more variety.
- Substitute the eggs with 1/4 cup of crumbled tofu for a vegan option.

11. Spicy Black Bean & Sweet Potato Buddha Bowl with Quinoa

This recipe offers a unique combination of flavor and textures while being well-tailored for diabetics:

Ingredients:

- 1 cup cooked quinoa (rinsed and drained)
- 1/2 cup mashed black beans (low-sodium)
- 1 medium sweet potato, roasted and diced
- 1/2 cup chopped romaine lettuce
- 1/4 cup chopped red onion
- 1/4 cup chopped bell pepper (any color)
- 1/4 cup cherry tomatoes, halved
- 1/4 cup crumbled feta cheese (optional)
- 1 tbsp olive oil
- 1 tsp lime juice
- 1/2 tsp chili powder
- 1/4 tsp cumin
- 1/4 tsp smoked paprika
- Pinch of salt and black pepper
- Cilantro leaves, for garnish (optional)

Instructions:

1. Preheat oven to 400°F (200°C). Dice sweet potato and toss with 1/2 tbsp olive oil and a pinch of salt. Roast for 20-25 minutes, or until tender.
2. While the sweet potato roasts, prepare the dressing by whisking together remaining olive oil, lime juice, chili powder, cumin, paprika, salt, and pepper.

3. Assemble the bowls by dividing quinoa, black beans, roasted sweet potato, lettuce, onion, bell pepper, and cherry tomatoes evenly between two bowls.
4. Top with crumbled feta cheese (optional) and drizzle with the prepared dressing.
5. Garnish with fresh cilantro leaves (optional) and enjoy!

Nutritional Information:

- Calories: 400
- Carbohydrates: 40g
- Fiber: 10g
- Protein: 15g
- Fat: 15g

Tips:

- Substitute quinoa with brown rice or barley for a different grain option.
- Use low-fat or fat-free feta cheese to reduce saturated fat content.
- Add a dollop of plain Greek yogurt for extra protein and creaminess.
- Adjust the spice level of the dressing to your preference.

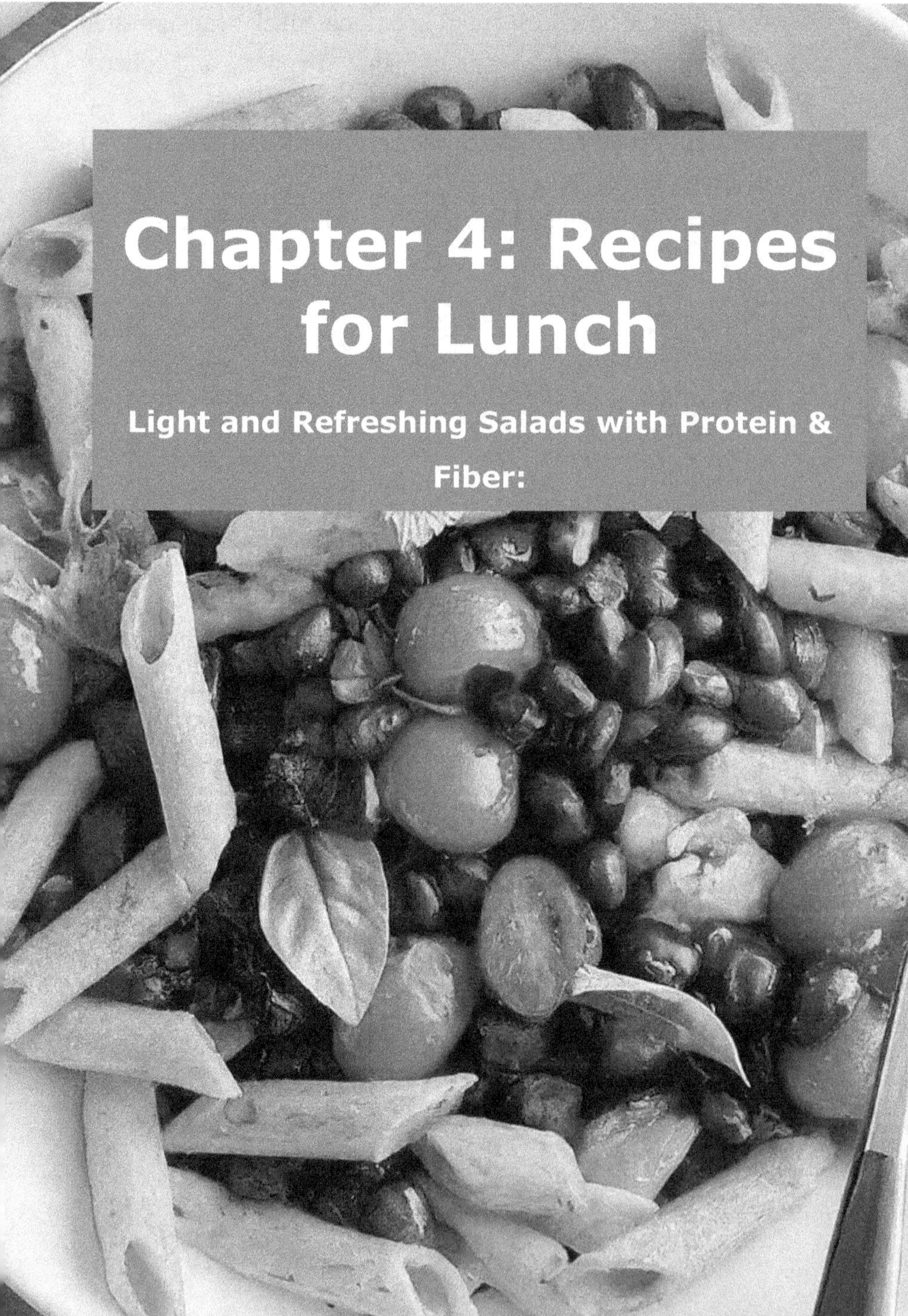
Chapter 4: Recipes for Lunch

Light and Refreshing Salads with Protein & Fiber:

Mediterranean Tuna Salad with Arugula, Olives, and Feta (Diabetic-Friendly):

Ingredients:

- 1 can (5 oz) water-packed tuna, flaked
- 2 cups baby arugula
- 1/2 cup cherry tomatoes, halved
- 1/4 cup kalamata olives, pitted and halved
- 1/4 cup crumbled feta cheese
- 1/4 cup red onion, diced
- 2 tbsp olive oil
- 1 tbsp lemon juice
- 1 tsp dried oregano
- Pinch of stevia (optional)
- 2 cups romaine lettuce leaves (for bed)

Instructions:

1. In a large bowl, combine tuna, arugula, tomatoes, olives, feta, and red onion.
2. In a small bowl, whisk together olive oil, lemon juice, oregano, and stevia (optional).
3. Pour dressing over salad and toss gently to coat.
4. Serve on a bed of romaine lettuce leaves and enjoy!

Nutritional Information:

- Calories: 350, Carbohydrates: 15g
- Fiber: 3g, Protein: 30g, Fat: 20g

Tips:

- Use low-sodium feta cheese to reduce salt intake.
- Substitute black beans for half the tuna for added fiber and protein.
- Add chopped cucumber or zucchini for extra volume and hydration.

Chicken Caesar Salad with Sprouts and Roasted Beets (Diabetic-Friendly):

Ingredients:

- 4 oz grilled chicken breast, sliced
- 2 cups romaine lettuce leaves
- 1 cup shaved Brussels sprouts
- 1/2 cup roasted diced beets
- 1/4 cup alfalfa sprouts
- 1/4 cup Caesar dressing (made with Greek yogurt, Dijon mustard, and stevia)
- 1 tbsp grated Parmesan cheese

Instructions:

1. In a large bowl, combine chicken, romaine, Brussels sprouts, beets, and sprouts.
2. Drizzle with Caesar dressing and toss gently to coat.
3. Top with Parmesan cheese and serve immediately.

Nutritional Information:

- Calories: 300
- Carbohydrates: 20g
- Fiber: 4g
- Protein: 30g
- Fat: 15g

Tips:

- Roast beets at home with minimal oil and a sprinkle of stevia for sweetness.
- Use a low-fat or fat-free Greek yogurt for the dressing.
- Add chopped walnuts or pecans for additional healthy fats.

Spicy Black Bean and Corn Salad with Cilantro Lime Dressing (Diabetic-Friendly):

Ingredients:

- 1 can (15 oz) black beans, rinsed and drained
- 1 can (15 oz) corn, rinsed and drained
- 1/2 cup bell pepper, chopped (any color)
- 1/4 cup red onion, chopped
- 2 cups romaine lettuce, chopped
- 1/4 cup chopped cilantro
- 1 jalapeno (optional, adjust for spice preference)
- 1/4 cup olive oil
- 2 tbsp lime juice
- 1 tsp cumin
- 1/2 tsp chili powder
- Pinch of stevia (optional)

Instructions:

1. In a large bowl, combine black beans, corn, bell pepper, red onion, romaine, and cilantro.
2. If using, finely chop the jalapeno and add to the bowl.
3. In a small bowl, whisk together olive oil, lime juice, cumin, chili powder, and stevia (optional).
4. Pour dressing over salad and toss gently to coat.
5. Serve immediately or refrigerate for later.

Nutritional Information:

- Calories: 300
- Carbohydrates: 35g
- Fiber: 8g
- Protein: 15g
- Fat: 10g

Tips:

- Use low-sodium canned beans to reduce salt intake.
- Substitute chickpeas for black beans for added protein.
- Add chopped avocado for a creamy texture and healthy fats.

One-Pot Meals for Busy Days:

Curried Lentil Soup with Spinach and Cauliflower (Diabetic-Friendly):

Ingredients:

- 1 cup green lentils, rinsed
- 4 cups vegetable broth (low-sodium)
- 1 can (13.5 oz) coconut milk, light
- 2 tbsp curry powder
- 1 head cauliflower, chopped
- 4 cups baby spinach
- 1 can (14.5 oz) diced tomatoes, undrained
- 1 inch ginger, grated (optional)
- Pinch of stevia (optional)
- Chopped cucumber and cilantro, for garnish

Instructions:

1. In a large pot, combine lentils, broth, coconut milk, curry powder, and cauliflower.
2. Bring to a boil, then reduce heat and simmer for 20-25 minutes, or until lentils are tender.
3. Add spinach and tomatoes, and cook for an additional 5 minutes, or until spinach is wilted.
4. Season with ginger (optional) and stevia (optional) to taste.
5. Serve hot, garnished with chopped cucumber and cilantro.

Nutritional Information:

- Calories: 300
- Carbohydrates: 40g
- Fiber: 10g
- Protein: 15g
- Fat: 15g

Tips:

- Use pre-washed and chopped cauliflower to save time.
- Substitute brown rice or quinoa for half the lentils for added texture and carbs.
- Omit the stevia if using sweetened coconut milk.

Salmon and Asparagus Stir-fry with Shiitake Mushrooms (Diabetic-Friendly):

Ingredients:

- 4 oz salmon fillet, skinless and boneless
- 1 tbsp sesame oil
- 1 tbsp reduced-sodium soy sauce
- 1 cup shiitake mushrooms, sliced
- 1 bunch asparagus, trimmed and cut into pieces
- 1 red bell pepper, sliced
- 1 clove garlic, minced
- 1 cup cooked brown rice or quinoa

Instructions:

1. Cut salmon into bite-sized pieces.
2. In a large skillet, heat sesame oil and soy sauce over medium-high heat.
3. Add salmon and cook for 3-4 minutes per side, or until cooked through.
4. Remove salmon from pan and set aside.
5. Add mushrooms, asparagus, and bell pepper to the pan and cook for 5-7 minutes, or until tender-crisp.
6. Add garlic and cook for an additional minute.
7. Return salmon to the pan and stir to combine.
8. Serve over cooked brown rice or quinoa.

Nutritional Information:

- Calories: 400
- Carbohydrates: 30g
- Fiber: 4g
- Protein: 35g
- Fat: 20g

Tips:

- Use low-sodium soy sauce to further reduce sodium content.
- Add other vegetables like broccoli or zucchini for more variety.
- Serve with a low-sugar dipping sauce, like low-sodium tamari or a drizzle of lemon juice.

Tuscan White Bean Soup with Kale and Sausage (Diabetic-Friendly):

Ingredients:

- 1 tbsp olive oil
- 1/2 lb Italian sausage (mild or sweet), links or ground
- 1 cup chopped kale
- 1 can (28 oz) diced tomatoes, undrained
- 1 can (15 oz) cannellini beans, rinsed and drained
- 4 cups vegetable broth (low-sodium)
- 1 clove garlic, minced
- 1 tsp dried oregano
- Black pepper to taste
- Pinch of stevia (optional)

Instructions:

1. In a large pot, heat olive oil over medium heat.
2. Add sausage and cook until browned, breaking it up into crumbles.
3. Add kale and cook for a few minutes, until wilted.
4. Stir in tomatoes, cannellini beans, broth, garlic, and oregano.
5. Bring to a boil, then reduce heat and simmer for 20-25 minutes, or until vegetables are tender.
6. Season with black pepper and stevia (optional) to taste.
7. Serve hot, with crusty bread for dipping (optional).

Nutritional Information:

- Calories: 400
- Carbohydrates: 45g
- Fiber: 10g
- Protein: 25g
- Fat: 20g

Tips:

- Use low-fat Italian sausage to reduce saturated fat content.
- Substitute white beans with chickpeas or lentils for additional protein.
- Add a pinch of red pepper flakes for a spicy kick.

Global-Inspired Dishes with Diabetic-Friendly Adjustments:

Thai Chicken Lettuce Wraps with Mango Salsa (Diabetic-Friendly):

Ingredients:

- 4 oz boneless, skinless chicken breasts, grilled or baked
- 1/4 cup unsweetened coconut milk
- 1 tbsp lime juice
- 1 tsp grated ginger
- 1/4 tsp red pepper flakes (optional)
- 1 romaine lettuce head, leaves separated
- 1 carrot, shredded
- 1 cucumber, sliced
- 1/4 cup chopped peanuts
- 1 mango, diced
- 1/4 red onion, finely chopped
- 1 tbsp chopped cilantro
- 1 tbsp lime juice
- Pinch of stevia (optional)

Instructions:

1. Marinate chicken in a mixture of coconut milk, lime juice, ginger, and red pepper flakes (optional) for at least 30 minutes.
2. Grill or bake chicken until cooked through.
3. Shred or slice chicken thinly.
4. Assemble lettuce wraps with chicken, shredded carrot, sliced cucumber, and chopped peanuts.

5. For the mango salsa, combine diced mango, red onion, cilantro, lime juice, and stevia (optional).
6. Top lettuce wraps with the mango salsa and enjoy!

Nutritional Information:

- Calories: 350
- Carbohydrates: 25g
- Fiber: 4g
- Protein: 30g
- Fat: 15g

Tips:

- Use low-fat coconut milk for reduced saturated fat content.
- Substitute tofu or tempeh for a vegetarian option.
- Add bell peppers or other chopped vegetables to the lettuce wraps for more variety.

Mediterranean Chicken Bowls with Roasted Vegetables and Hummus (Diabetic-Friendly):

Ingredients:

- 4 oz boneless, skinless chicken breast, grilled or baked
- 1 zucchini, diced
- 1 eggplant, diced
- 1 red bell pepper, sliced
- 1 red onion, sliced
- 1 tbsp olive oil
- 1 tsp dried oregano
- Salt and pepper to taste
- 4 cups romaine lettuce, chopped
- 1 cucumber, chopped
- 1/4 cup cherry tomatoes, halved
- 1/4 cup kalamata olives, pitted and halved
- 1/4 cup reduced-fat hummus

Instructions:

1. Preheat oven to 400°F (200°C).
2. Toss zucchini, eggplant, bell pepper, and onion with olive oil, oregano, salt, and pepper.
3. Roast vegetables for 20-25 minutes, or until tender.
4. Slice or shred chicken.
5. Assemble bowls with romaine lettuce, chopped cucumber, cherry tomatoes, olives, roasted vegetables, and chicken.
6. Top with a dollop of reduced-fat hummus and enjoy!

Nutritional Information:

- Calories: 400
- Carbohydrates: 30g
- Fiber: 8g
- Protein: 35g
- Fat: 20g

Tips:

- Use lean ground turkey or chicken breast for a lower-fat option.
- Roast other vegetables like broccoli or asparagus for variety.
- Make your own hummus using canned chickpeas, tahini, lemon juice, and spices.

Indian Spiced Chickpea Curry with Cauliflower Rice (Diabetic-Friendly):

Ingredients:

- 1 tbsp olive oil
- 1 onion, chopped
- 1 clove garlic, minced
- 1 tsp ground cumin
- 1/2 tsp turmeric
- 1/4 tsp ground coriander
- 1 can (14.5 oz) diced tomatoes, undrained
- 1 cup water
- 1 can (15 oz) chickpeas, rinsed and drained
- 1 head cauliflower, chopped
- Pinch of stevia (optional)
- Chopped cilantro, for garnish

Instructions:

1. Heat olive oil in a large pot over medium heat.
2. Add onion and cook until softened, about 5 minutes.
3. Add garlic, cumin, turmeric, and coriander, and cook for 1 minute more.
4. Stir in diced tomatoes, water, and chickpeas.
5. Bring to a boil, then reduce heat and simmer for 15 minutes.
6. While the curry simmers, pulse cauliflower in a food processor until it resembles rice.
7. Steam or boil cauliflower rice until tender.
8. Season the curry with stevia (optional) to taste.
9. Serve curry over cauliflower rice and garnish with cilantro.

Nutritional Information:

- Calories: 300
- Carbohydrates: 40g
- Fiber: 10g
- Protein: 15g
- Fat: 10g

Tips:

- Use low-sodium diced tomatoes to further reduce sodium content.
- Substitute brown rice or quinoa for cauliflower rice for added texture and protein.
- Add other vegetables like spinach or bell peppers for more variety.

Hearty and Comforting Options:

Baked Salmon with Roasted Brussels Sprouts and Sweet Potato Mash (Diabetic-Friendly):

Ingredients:

- 4 oz salmon fillet, skinless and boneless
- 1 tbsp olive oil
- 1/2 tsp dried thyme
- Salt and pepper to taste
- 1 cup Brussels sprouts, trimmed and halved
- 1 sweet potato, peeled and diced
- 1/4 cup unsweetened almond milk
- Pinch of stevia (optional)

Instructions:

1. Preheat oven to 400°F (200°C).
2. Toss salmon with olive oil, thyme, salt, and pepper.
3. Place salmon on a baking sheet lined with parchment paper.
4. Roast for 15-20 minutes, or until cooked through.
5. While the salmon cooks, roast Brussels sprouts on a separate baking sheet for 20-25 minutes, or until tender-crisp.
6. Boil sweet potato chunks until tender.
7. Mash sweet potato with almond milk and stevia (optional) to taste.
8. Serve salmon with roasted Brussels sprouts and sweet potato mash.

Nutritional Information:

- Calories: 400
- Carbohydrates: 35g
- Fiber: 8g
- Protein: 30g
- Fat: 20g

Tips:

- Use low-sodium soy sauce or tamari instead of salt for a different flavor profile.
- Substitute white potatoes for sweet potatoes, adjusting stevia accordingly.
- Add a dollop of low-fat Greek yogurt to the sweet potato mash for extra protein.

Turkey Chili with Kidney Beans and Corn (Diabetic-Friendly):

Ingredients:

- 1 tbsp olive oil
- 1/2 lb ground turkey (lean)
- 1 onion, chopped
- 1 clove garlic, minced
- 1 green bell pepper, chopped
- 1 can (15 oz) kidney beans, rinsed and drained
- 1 can (15 oz) diced tomatoes, undrained
- 1 can (15 oz) corn, rinsed and drained
- 4 cups vegetable broth (low-sodium)
- 1 tbsp chili powder
- 1 tsp cumin
- 1/2 tsp smoked paprika
- Salt and pepper to taste
- Chopped avocado and cilantro, for garnish (optional)

Instructions:

1. Heat olive oil in a large pot over medium heat.
2. Brown ground turkey, breaking it up with a spoon.
3. Add onion, garlic, and bell pepper, and cook until softened, about 5 minutes.
4. Stir in kidney beans, diced tomatoes, corn, broth, chili powder, cumin, paprika, salt, and pepper.
5. Bring to a boil, then reduce heat and simmer for 30 minutes, or until chili is thickened and flavors are melded.
6. Serve chili hot, garnished with chopped avocado and cilantro (optional).

Nutritional Information:

- Calories: 400
- Carbohydrates: 45g
- Fiber: 10g
- Protein: 30g
- Fat: 20g

Tips:

- Use black beans instead of kidney beans for added protein.
- Substitute ground chicken or lentils for turkey for different protein options.
- Adjust the spice level by adding more or less chili powder.

Lentil Shepherd's Pie with Cauliflower Mash (Diabetic-Friendly):

Ingredients:

- 1 tbsp olive oil
- 1 onion, chopped
- 1 carrot, chopped
- 1 celery stalk, chopped
- 1 cup green lentils, rinsed
- 4 cups vegetable broth (low-sodium)
- 1 can (15 oz) diced tomatoes, undrained
- 1/2 cup frozen peas
- 1/4 cup frozen corn
- 1 head cauliflower, chopped
- 1/4 cup unsweetened almond milk
- Pinch of stevia (optional)

Instructions:

1. Heat olive oil in a large pot over medium heat.
2. Sauté onion, carrot, and celery until softened, about 5 minutes.
3. Add lentils, broth, and diced tomatoes to the pot.
4. Bring to a boil, then reduce heat and simmer for 20-25 minutes, or until lentils are tender.
5. Stir in frozen peas and corn, and cook for an additional 5 minutes.
6. Preheat oven to 400°F (200°C).
7. While the lentil mixture cooks, steam or boil cauliflower florets until tender.
8. Mash cauliflower with almond milk and stevia (optional) until smooth.

9. Transfer the lentil mixture to a baking dish.

10. Top with cauliflower mash, spreading it evenly.

11. Bake for 20-225 minutes, or until the mash is golden brown and the filling is bubbly.

Nutritional Information:

- Calories: 350
- Carbohydrates: 40g
- Fiber: 12g
- Protein: 15g
- Fat: 15g

Tips:

- Use low-sodium vegetable broth to further reduce sodium content.
- Substitute brown rice or quinoa for half the lentils for added texture and protein.
- Add other vegetables like chopped mushrooms or spinach to the lentil mixture for more variety.

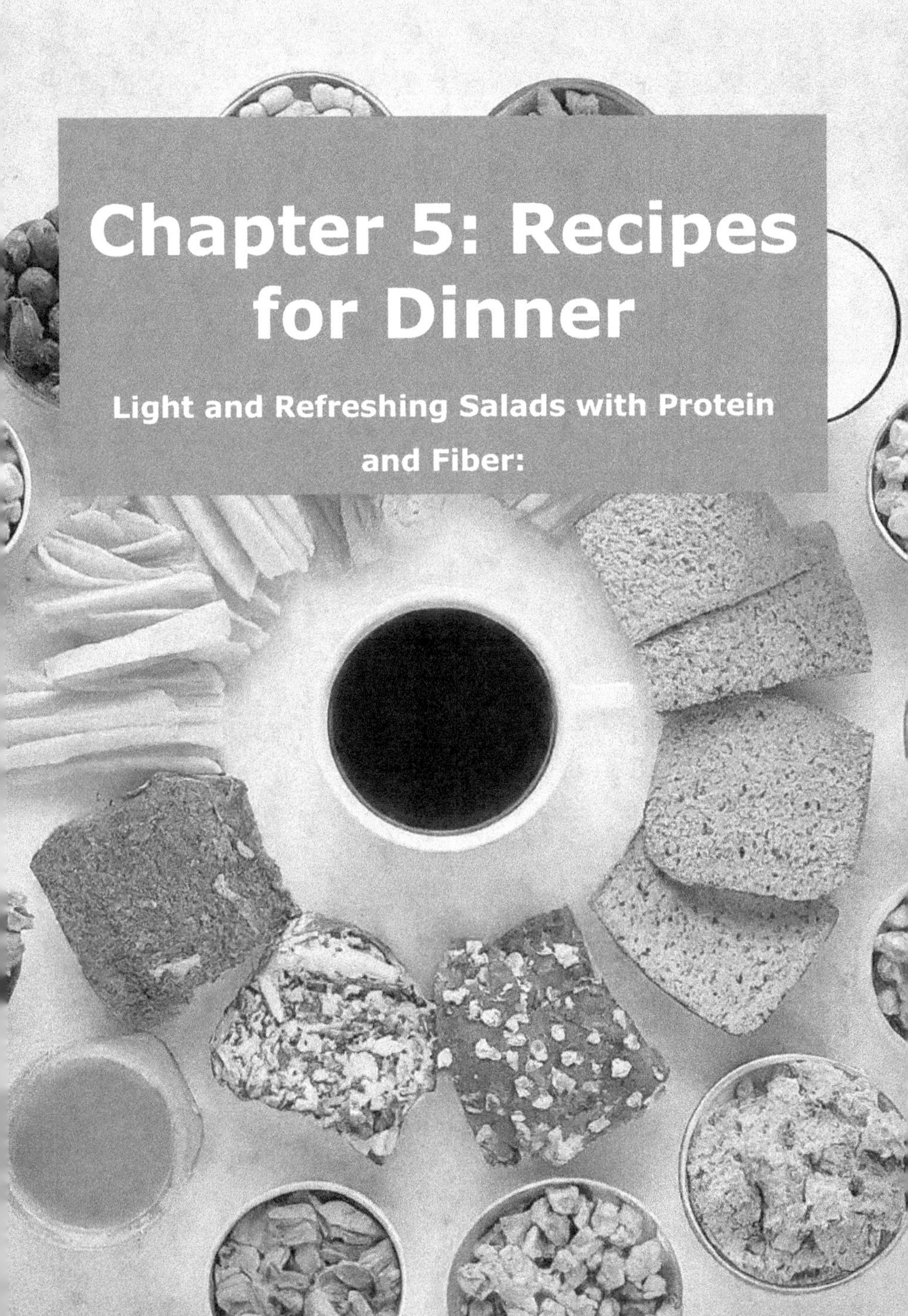

Chapter 5: Recipes for Dinner
Light and Refreshing Salads with Protein and Fiber:

Mediterranean Tuna Salad with White Beans and Arugula (Diabetic-Friendly):

Ingredients:

- 1 can (5 oz) water-packed tuna, flaked
- 1/2 cup cooked cannellini beans, rinsed and drained
- 1/2 cup chopped cucumber
- 1/2 cup chopped cherry tomatoes
- 1/4 cup Kalamata olives, pitted and halved
- 1/4 cup red onion, diced
- 1/4 cup crumbled feta cheese (reduced-fat)
- 2 tbsp olive oil
- 1 tbsp lemon juice
- 1 clove garlic, minced
- 1/2 tsp dried oregano
- 2 cups baby arugula leaves

Instructions:

1. In a large bowl, combine tuna, cannellini beans, cucumber, tomatoes, olives, red onion, and feta cheese.
2. In a small bowl, whisk together olive oil, lemon juice, garlic, and oregano.
3. Pour dressing over the salad and toss gently to coat.
4. Serve on a bed of arugula leaves.

Nutritional Information:
- Calories: 350
- Carbohydrates: 25g
- Fiber: 12g
- Protein: 20g
- Fat: 20g

Tips:

- Use low-sodium canned beans and feta cheese to reduce sodium intake.
- Substitute chickpeas for half the white beans for added protein and fiber.
- Add chopped bell peppers or celery for more variety.

Salmon Nicoise Salad with Asparagus and Eggs (Diabetic-Friendly):

Ingredients:

- 4 oz salmon fillet, skinless and boneless
- 2 cups mixed greens
- 1/2 cup asparagus tips, blanched
- 2 hard-boiled eggs, sliced
- 1/4 cup cherry tomatoes, halved
- 1/4 cup Kalamata olives, pitted and halved
- 1/4 cup green beans, steamed or blanched
- 2 tbsp Dijon mustard
- 1 tbsp olive oil
- 1 tbsp lemon juice
- 1/4 tsp dried dill
- Salt and pepper to taste

Instructions:

1. Pan-sear salmon according to desired doneness.
2. Arrange mixed greens on a plate.
3. Top with asparagus tips, hard-boiled eggs, cherry tomatoes, olives, and green beans.
4. In a small bowl, whisk together Dijon mustard, olive oil, lemon juice, and dill.
5. Drizzle dressing over the salad and top with flaked salmon.
6. Season with salt and pepper to taste.

Nutritional Information:

- Calories: 350
- Carbohydrates: 20g
- Fiber: 5g
- Protein: 25g
- Fat: 22g

Tips:

- Use low-fat yogurt substitute for mayonnaise in the Dijon dressing.
- Substitute grilled chicken or shrimp for the salmon for a different protein option.
- Add chopped avocado for healthy fats and creaminess.

Spicy Thai Chicken Salad with Peanut Dressing (Diabetic-Friendly):

Ingredients:

- 4 oz cooked chicken breast, shredded
- 1 carrot, shredded
- 1 red bell pepper, julienned
- 1 cucumber, julienned
- 1/4 cup chopped cilantro
- 2 green onions, sliced
- 1 tbsp unsweetened peanut butter
- 1 tbsp soy sauce (reduced-sodium)
- 1 tbsp lime juice
- 1 tsp Sriracha (adjust for spice preference)
- 1/4 cup water

Instructions:

1. In a large bowl, combine chicken, carrot, bell pepper, cucumber, cilantro, and green onions.
2. In a small bowl, whisk together peanut butter, soy sauce, lime juice, Sriracha, and water until smooth.
3. Pour dressing over the salad and toss gently to coat.

Nutritional Information:

- Calories: 300
- Carbohydrates: 20g
- Fiber: 5g
- Protein: 22g
- Fat: 15g

Tips:

- Use low-sodium soy sauce to further reduce sodium content.
- Substitute tofu or tempeh for the chicken for a vegetarian option.
- Add chopped cashews or peanuts for extra protein and crunch.

One-Pot Meals for Busy Days:

Salmon and Veggie Stir-Fry with Quinoa (Diabetic-Friendly):

Ingredients:

- 4 oz salmon fillet, skinless and boneless
- 1 tbsp sesame oil
- 1 tbsp reduced-sodium soy sauce
- 1 cup broccoli florets
- 1 bell pepper, sliced
- 1/2 cup snow peas
- 1 clove garlic, minced
- 1 cup cooked quinoa

Instructions:

1. Cut salmon into bite-sized pieces.
2. In a large skillet, heat sesame oil and soy sauce over medium-high heat.
3. Add salmon and cook for 3-4 minutes per side, or until cooked through.
4. Remove salmon from pan and set aside.
5. Add broccoli, bell pepper, and snow peas to the pan and cook for 5-7 minutes, or until tender-crisp.
6. Add garlic and cook for an additional minute.
7. Return salmon to the pan and stir to combine.
8. Serve over cooked quinoa.

Nutritional Information:

- Calories: 400
- Carbohydrates: 30g
- Fiber: 4g
- Protein: 35g
- Fat: 20g

Tips:

- Use low-sodium soy sauce to further reduce sodium content.
- Add other vegetables like mushrooms or carrots for more variety.
- Serve with a low-sugar dipping sauce, like low-sodium tamari or a drizzle of lemon juice.

One-Pot Mediterranean Chicken and Vegetable Pasta (Diabetic-Friendly):

Ingredients:

- 1 tbsp olive oil
- 1 boneless, skinless chicken breast, sliced
- 1 zucchini, diced
- 1 cup cherry tomatoes, halved
- 1/4 cup Kalamata olives, pitted and halved
- 1 cup whole-wheat pasta
- 4 cups chicken broth (low-sodium)
- 1 tsp dried oregano
- Salt and pepper to taste

Instructions:

1. In a large pot, heat olive oil over medium heat.
2. Add chicken and cook until browned on both sides.
3. Add zucchini, tomatoes, and olives to the pot.
4. Stir in pasta, chicken broth, and oregano.
5. Bring to a boil, then reduce heat and simmer for 15-20 minutes, or until pasta is cooked through and vegetables are tender.
6. Season with salt and pepper to taste.

Nutritional Information:

- Calories: 450
- Carbohydrates: 45g
- Fiber: 8g
- Protein: 30g
- Fat: 18g

Tips:

- Use whole-wheat pasta for added fiber and nutrients.
- Substitute shrimp or lentils for the chicken for different protein options.
- Add a sprinkle of Parmesan cheese for extra flavor.

Global-Inspired Dishes with Diabetic-Friendly Adjustments:

Mediterranean Chicken Bowls with Roasted Vegetables and Hummus (Diabetic-Friendly):

Ingredients:

- 4 oz boneless, skinless chicken breast, grilled or baked
- 1 tbsp olive oil
- 1/2 tsp dried oregano
- Salt and pepper to taste
- 1 head cauliflower, chopped
- 1 red onion, sliced
- 1 red bell pepper, sliced
- 1 can (15 oz) chickpeas, rinsed and drained
- 1/4 cup reduced-fat hummus
- Chopped cucumber, cherry tomatoes, and cilantro, for garnish

Instructions:

1. Preheat oven to 400°F (200°C).
2. Toss chicken with olive oil, oregano, salt, and pepper.
3. Grill or bake the chicken until cooked through.
4. While the chicken cooks, toss cauliflower, onion, and bell pepper with olive oil and spread on a baking sheet.
5. Roast for 20-25 minutes, or until tender-crisp.
6. To assemble bowls, divide roasted vegetables, chickpeas, and chopped cucumber and tomatoes among bowls.
7. Add sliced or shredded chicken and top with a dollop of hummus.
8. Garnish with fresh cilantro if desired.

Nutritional Information:

- Calories: 400
- Carbohydrates: 30g
- Fiber: 10g
- Protein: 30g
- Fat: 20g

Tips:

- Use low-sodium chicken broth for marinating the chicken to further reduce sodium content.
- Substitute tofu or tempeh for the chicken for a vegetarian option.
- Add other roasted vegetables like broccoli or zucchini for more variety.
- Make your own hummus using canned chickpeas, tahini, lemon juice, and spices for more control over ingredients.

Indian Chickpea Curry with Cauliflower Rice (Diabetic-Friendly):

Ingredients:

- 1 tbsp olive oil
- 1 onion, chopped
- 1 clove garlic, minced
- 1 tsp ground cumin
- 1/2 tsp turmeric
- 1/4 tsp ground coriander
- 1 can (14.5 oz) diced tomatoes, undrained
- 1 cup water
- 1 can (15 oz) chickpeas, rinsed and drained
- 1 head cauliflower, chopped
- Pinch of stevia (optional)
- Chopped cilantro, for garnish

Instructions:

1. Heat olive oil in a large pot over medium heat.
2. Add onion and cook until softened, about 5 minutes.
3. Add garlic, cumin, turmeric, and coriander, and cook for 1 minute more.
4. Stir in diced tomatoes, water, and chickpeas.
5. Bring to a boil, then reduce heat and simmer for 15 minutes.
6. While the curry simmers, pulse cauliflower in a food processor until it resembles rice.
7. Steam or boil cauliflower rice until tender.
8. Season the curry with stevia (optional) to taste.
9. Serve curry over cauliflower rice and garnish with chopped cilantro.

Nutritional Information:

- Calories: 300
- Carbohydrates: 40g
- Fiber: 12g
- Protein: 15g
- Fat: 10g

Tips:

- Use low-sodium diced tomatoes to further reduce sodium content.
- Substitute brown rice or quinoa for cauliflower rice for added texture and protein.
- Add other vegetables like spinach or bell peppers for more variety.

Thai Lettuce Wraps with Shrimp and Peanut Sauce (Diabetic-Friendly):

Ingredients:

- 4 oz shrimp, peeled and deveined
- 1 tbsp olive oil
- 1/2 tsp garlic powder
- 1/4 tsp ground ginger
- 1 bell pepper, julienned
- 1 carrot, julienned
- 1 cucumber, julienned
- 1/4 cup chopped cilantro
- 1/4 cup chopped green onions
- 1 romaine lettuce head, leaves separated

Peanut Sauce:

- 1 tbsp unsweetened peanut butter
- 1 tbsp soy sauce (reduced-sodium)
- 1 tbsp lime juice
- 1 tsp Sriracha (adjust for spice preference)
- 1/4 cup water

Instructions:

1. Marinate shrimp in olive oil, garlic powder, and ginger for 15 minutes.
2. Cook shrimp in a pan or grill until cooked through.
3. Prepare vegetables and assemble lettuce wraps with shrimp, bell pepper, carrot, cucumber, cilantro, and green onions.
4. In a small bowl, whisk together peanut butter, soy sauce, lime juice, Sriracha, and water until smooth. Adjust the Sriracha amount to your desired spice level.

5. Drizzle peanut sauce over the lettuce wraps and enjoy!

Nutritional Information:

- Calories: 300
- Carbohydrates: 20g
- Fiber: 5g
- Protein: 25g
- Fat: 15g

Tips:

- Use low-sodium soy sauce to further reduce sodium content.
- Substitute tofu or tempeh for the shrimp for a vegetarian option.
- Add chopped peanuts or cashews for extra protein and crunch.
- Serve with additional lime wedges for squeezing over the wraps.

Hearty and Comforting Options:

Baked Salmon with Roasted Brussels Sprouts and Quinoa (Diabetic-Friendly):

Ingredients:

- 4 oz salmon fillet, skinless and boneless
- 1 tbsp olive oil
- 1/2 tsp dried thyme
- Salt and pepper to taste
- 1 cup Brussels sprouts, trimmed and halved
- 1 cup cooked quinoa
- 1/4 cup sliced almonds, toasted (optional)
- Lemon wedges, for garnish

Instructions:

1. Preheat oven to 400°F (200°C).
2. Toss salmon with olive oil, thyme, salt, and pepper.
3. Place salmon on a baking sheet lined with parchment paper.
4. Roast for 15-20 minutes, or until cooked through.
5. While the salmon cooks, toss Brussels sprouts with olive oil and spread on a separate baking sheet.
6. Roast for 20-25 minutes, or until tender-crisp.
7. Serve salmon with roasted Brussels sprouts and quinoa. Garnish with toasted almonds (optional) and lemon wedges.

Nutritional Information:

- Calories: 400
- Carbohydrates: 35g
- Fiber: 8g
- Protein: 32g
- Fat: 20g

Tips:

- Use low-sodium soy sauce or tamari instead of salt for a different flavor profile.
- Substitute white potatoes for quinoa, adjusting stevia accordingly.
- Add a dollop of low-fat Greek yogurt to the quinoa for extra protein.

Lentil Shepherd's Pie with Mashed Cauliflower (Diabetic-Friendly):

Ingredients:

- 1 tbsp olive oil
- 1/2 lb ground turkey (lean)
- 1 onion, chopped
- 1 clove garlic, minced
- 1 green bell pepper, chopped
- 1 cup green lentils, rinsed
- 4 cups vegetable broth (low-sodium)
- 1 can (15 oz) diced tomatoes, undrained
- 1 cup frozen peas
- 1/2 cup frozen corn
- 1 head cauliflower, chopped
- 1/4 cup unsweetened almond milk
- Pinch of stevia (optional)

Instructions:

1. Heat olive oil in a large pot over medium heat.
2. Brown ground turkey, breaking it up with a spoon.
3. Add onion, garlic, and bell pepper, and cook until softened, about 5 minutes.
4. Stir in lentils, broth, diced tomatoes, peas, and corn.
5. Bring to a boil, then reduce heat and simmer for 20-25 minutes, or until lentils are tender and the mixture is thickened.
6. While the lentil mixture cooks, steam or boil cauliflower florets until tender.
7. Mash cauliflower with almond milk and stevia (optional) until smooth.

8. Preheat oven to 400°F (200°C).
9. Transfer the lentil mixture to a baking dish.
10. Top with cauliflower mash, spreading it evenly.
11. Bake for 20-25 minutes, or until the mash is golden brown and the filling is bubbly.

Nutritional Information:

- Calories: 350
- Carbohydrates: 40g
- Fiber: 15g
- Protein: 20g
- Fat: 15g

Tips:

- Use low-sodium vegetable broth to further reduce sodium content.
- Substitute brown rice or quinoa for half the lentils for added texture and protein.
- Add other vegetables like chopped mushrooms or spinach to the lentil mixture for more variety.

Turkey Chili with Black Beans and Sweet Potato (Diabetic-Friendly):

Ingredients:

- 1 tbsp olive oil
- 1/2 lb ground turkey (lean)
- 1 onion, chopped
- 1 clove garlic, minced
- 1 green bell pepper, chopped
- 1 can (15 oz) black beans, rinsed and drained
- 1 can (15 oz) diced tomatoes, undrained
- 1 can (14.5 oz) diced sweet potatoes, undrained
- 4 cups vegetable broth (low-sodium)
- 1 tbsp chili powder
- 1 tsp cumin
- 1/2 tsp smoked paprika
- Salt and pepper to taste
- Chopped avocado and cilantro, for garnish (optional)

Instructions:

1. Heat olive oil in a large pot over medium heat.
2. Brown ground turkey, breaking it up with a spoon.
3. Add onion, garlic, and bell pepper, and cook until softened, about 5 minutes.
4. Stir in black beans, diced tomatoes, diced sweet potatoes, vegetable broth, chili powder, cumin, and smoked paprika.
5. Bring to a boil, then reduce heat and simmer for 20-25 minutes, or until the sweet potatoes are tender and the chili has thickened.
6. Season with salt and pepper to taste.

7. Serve hot, garnished with chopped avocado and cilantro (optional).

Nutritional Information:

- Calories: 400
- Carbohydrates: 40g
- Fiber: 12g
- Protein: 28g
- Fat: 20g

Tips:

- Use low-sodium canned beans, diced tomatoes, and vegetable broth to further reduce sodium content.
- Substitute ground chicken or ground beef for the ground turkey.
- Add other vegetables like corn, zucchini, or chopped mushrooms for more variety.
- Serve with a side of whole-wheat bread or brown rice for a complete meal.

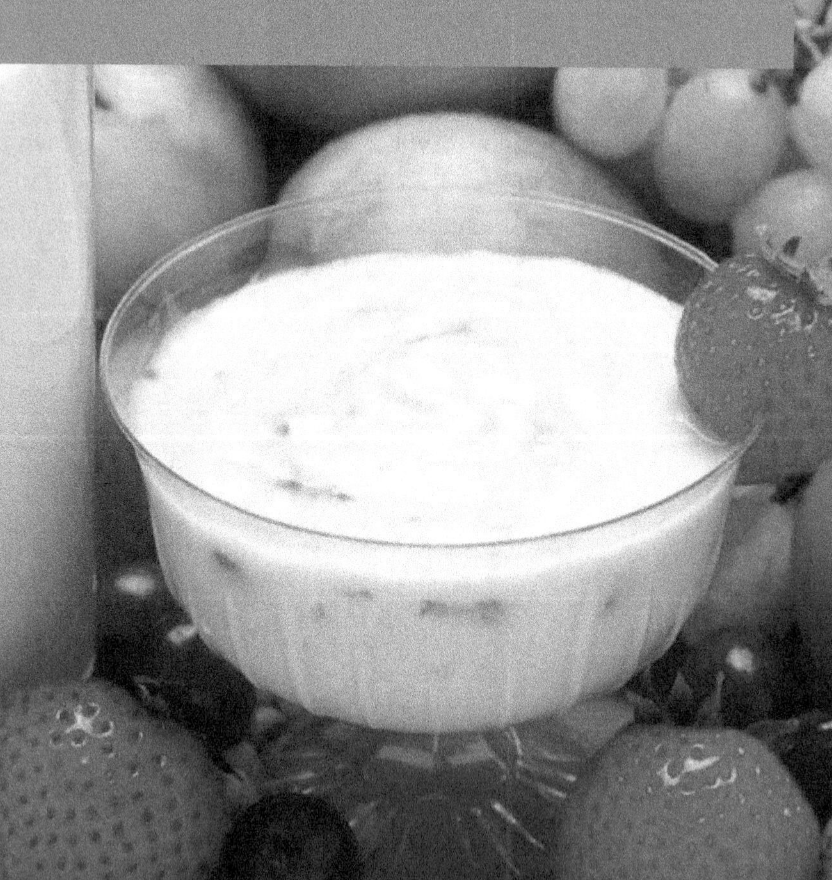

Chapter 6: Creative Snacks and Sides

Diabetic-Friendly Snacks and Sides:

Healthy Alternatives to Chips and Crackers:

Air-Fried Edamame Pods:

Ingredients:

1 cup frozen edamame pods, shelled

1/2 tsp Cajun seasoning (low-sodium) or nutritional yeast

Instructions:

1. Preheat your air fryer to 400°F (200°C).
2. Toss the edamame pods with your chosen seasoning.
3. Spread the seasoned edamame in a single layer in the air fryer basket.
4. Air-fry for 8-10 minutes, or until crispy and heated through.
5. Let cool slightly before enjoying.

Nutritional Information: (per serving)

- Calories: 120
- Carbohydrates: 14g
- Fiber: 8g
- Protein: 11g
- Fat: 6g

Tips:

- For a milder flavor, use paprika or garlic powder instead of Cajun seasoning.
- Experiment with different herbs and spices to find your favorite combination.
- Don't overcrowd the air fryer basket, as this can prevent the edamame from crisping evenly.

Roasted Beet Chips:

Ingredients:

- 2 medium beets, trimmed and thinly sliced (use a mandoline for even slices)
    - 1 tbsp olive oil
    - 1/2 tsp dried thyme
    - 1/4 tsp garlic powder
    - Salt and pepper to taste

Instructions:

1. Preheat oven to 400°F (200°C).
2. Line a baking sheet with parchment paper.
3. Toss the beet slices with olive oil, thyme, garlic powder, salt, and pepper.
4. Spread the seasoned beets in a single layer on the prepared baking sheet.
5. Roast for 20-25 minutes, or until the beets are tender and crispy around the edges.
6. Let cool completely before enjoying.

Nutritional Information: (per serving)

- Calories: 40
- Carbohydrates: 8g
- Fiber: 2g
- Protein: 1g
- Fat: 2g

Tips:

Use different colored beets for variety and visual appeal. Sprinkle the roasted chips with a touch of balsamic vinegar for an extra flavor boost.
Be sure the beets are sliced thinly to ensure even crisping.

Celery Sticks with Guacamole:

Ingredients:

- 2 celery stalks, cut into sticks
- 1/2 ripe avocado, mashed
- 1 tbsp lime juice
- 1/4 cup chopped tomato
- 1/4 cup chopped red onion
- 1/4 tsp chili powder
- Salt and pepper to taste

Instructions:

1. Mash the avocado with lime juice in a bowl.
2. Stir in the chopped tomato, onion, chili powder, salt, and pepper.
3. Serve the guacamole with celery sticks for dipping.

Nutritional Information: (per serving)

- Calories: 150
- Carbohydrates: 12g
- Fiber: 5g
- Protein: 4g
- Fat: 10g

- For a creamier guacamole, add a tablespoon of low-fat Greek yogurt.
- Sprinkle the guacamole with chopped cilantro for extra flavor.
- Use baby carrots or cucumber slices instead of celery for a different option.

Fruit-based Snacks with Protein and Fiber:

Greek Yogurt Parfait with Berries and Granola:

Ingredients:

- 1/2 cup plain Greek yogurt
- 1/4 cup mixed berries
- 1/4 cup sliced almonds
- 1 tbsp sugar-free granola

Instructions:

1. Layer the yogurt, berries, almonds, and granola in a parfait glass or bowl.
2. Enjoy immediately or refrigerate for later.

Nutritional Information: (per serving)

- Calories: 200
- Carbohydrates: 20g
- Fiber: 5g
- Protein: 15g
- Fat: 6g

Tips:

1. Use unsweetened or stevia-sweetened Greek yogurt to manage sugar intake.
2. Experiment with different fruits like melon, mango, or kiwi.
3. Choose a granola low in sugar and added sweeteners.

Apple "Nachos" with Nut Butter and Seeds:

Ingredients:

1 medium apple, thinly sliced
2 tbsp almond butter or other nut butter (unsweetened or sugar-free)
1/4 cup chia seeds
1/4 cup chopped walnuts
Optional: Drizzle of honey or sugar-free syrup

Instructions:

Arrange the apple slices on a plate or platter.
1. Dollop the nut butter evenly over the apple slices.
2. Sprinkle with chia seeds and chopped walnuts for added protein and texture.
3. If desired, drizzle with a small amount of honey or sugar-free syrup for a touch of sweetness.

Nutritional Information: (per serving)

- Calories: 250
- Carbohydrates: 30g
- Fiber: 6g
- Protein: 5g
- Fat: 15g

Tips:

- Use different types of apples for variety, such as Granny Smith, Honeycrisp, or Fuji.
- Toast the chopped walnuts for a deeper flavor.
- Substitute other seeds like pumpkin seeds or sunflower seeds for chia seeds.
- For a creamier topping, blend the nut butter with a tablespoon of unsweetened Greek yogurt.
- Add a sprinkle of cinnamon or nutmeg for extra warmth and flavor.

Sweet Treats that Satisfy without Spiking Blood Sugar:

Frozen Yogurt Bark with Berries and Nuts:

Ingredients:

1 cup plain Greek yogurt
1/4 cup stevia powder or other sugar-free sweetener
1/2 cup mixed berries, frozen
1/4 cup chopped nuts, toasted

Instructions:

Line a baking sheet with parchment paper.
In a bowl, whisk together the Greek yogurt and stevia powder until smooth.
Spread the yogurt mixture evenly onto the prepared baking sheet.
Sprinkle the frozen berries and chopped nuts over the yogurt layer.
Freeze for at least 2 hours, or until solid.
Break the frozen bark into pieces and enjoy.

Nutritional Information: (per serving)

- Calories: 150
- Carbohydrates: 16g
- Fiber: 3g
- Protein: 10g
- Fat: 5g

Tips:

- Use different types of berries for variety and color.
- Experiment with other toppings like chopped dark chocolate, shredded coconut, or sugar-free granola.
- Drizzle the bark with a touch of melted sugar-free chocolate for an extra treat.
- Make sure the berries are frozen to prevent them from sinking into the yogurt layer.

Roasted Pears with Ricotta and Spices:

Ingredients:

- 2 ripe pears, halved and cored
- 1/2 tsp ground cinnamon
- 1/4 tsp ground nutmeg
- 1/4 tsp ground cardamom
- 1/4 cup ricotta cheese
- 1 tablespoon honey (optional)

Instructions:

1. Preheat oven to 375°F (190°C).
2. In a small bowl, combine the cinnamon, nutmeg, and cardamom.
3. Sprinkle the spice mixture evenly over the cut sides of the pears.
4. Place the pears on a baking sheet lined with parchment paper.
5. Bake for 20-25 minutes, or until the pears are tender and starting to brown.
6. While the pears are baking, mix the ricotta cheese with honey (optional) in a small bowl.
7. Fill the cavities of the roasted pears with the ricotta cheese mixture.
8. Serve warm and enjoy.

Nutritional Information: (per serving)

- Calories: 200
- Carbohydrates: 30g
- Fiber: 5g
- Protein: 5g
- Fat: 5g

Tips:

1. Use different types of pears for variety, such as Bartlett, Bosc, or Anjou.
2. Drizzle the pears with a touch of maple syrup or balsamic vinegar for a different flavor profile.
3. Top the ricotta cheese with a sprinkle of chopped nuts or dried fruit for added texture and nutrients.
4. You can also grill the pears instead of roasting them for a smoky flavor.

Cucumber Slices with Cottage Cheese and Dill:

Ingredients:

- 1 cucumber, thinly sliced
- 1/2 cup low-fat cottage cheese
- 1 tablespoon fresh dill, chopped
- Pinch of black pepper
- Optional: Fresh mint leaves, for garnish

Instructions:

1. Arrange the cucumber slices on a plate or platter.
2. Dollop the cottage cheese evenly over the cucumber slices.
3. Sprinkle with chopped dill and black pepper.
4. Garnish with fresh mint leaves, if desired.

Nutritional Information: (per serving)

- Calories: 80
- Carbohydrates: 7g
- Fiber: 1g
- Protein: 6g
- Fat: 1g

Tips:

1. Use a mandoline slicer to get evenly thin cucumber slices.
2. Experiment with different fresh herbs like chives, parsley, or basil.
3. Add a dollop of low-fat sour cream or plain yogurt for additional creaminess.
4. Season with a squeeze of lemon juice for a touch of acidity.

Hard-boiled Eggs with Edamame Pods:

Ingredients:

- 4 eggs
- 1 cup frozen edamame pods, shelled
- Pinch of salt
- Black pepper to taste

Instructions:

1. Place the eggs in a saucepan and cover with cold water. Bring to a boil over medium heat.
2. Once boiling, remove from heat, cover, and let sit for 10-12 minutes for soft-boiled or 15-17 minutes for hard-boiled eggs.
3. Meanwhile, cook the edamame pods according to package directions.
4. Peel the eggs and enjoy with the edamame pods sprinkled with salt and pepper.

Nutritional Information: (per serving)

- Calories: 200
- Carbohydrates: 7g
- Fiber: 5g
- Protein: 17g
- Fat: 9g

- *Tips:*

- Use an ice bath to quickly cool the eggs after cooking to prevent overcooking.
- Peel the eggs under cold running water for easier removal of the shell.
- Sprinkle the edamame pods with your favorite spices like paprika, garlic powder, or chili flakes.
- Add chopped bell peppers, celery, or carrots for additional crunch and nutrients.

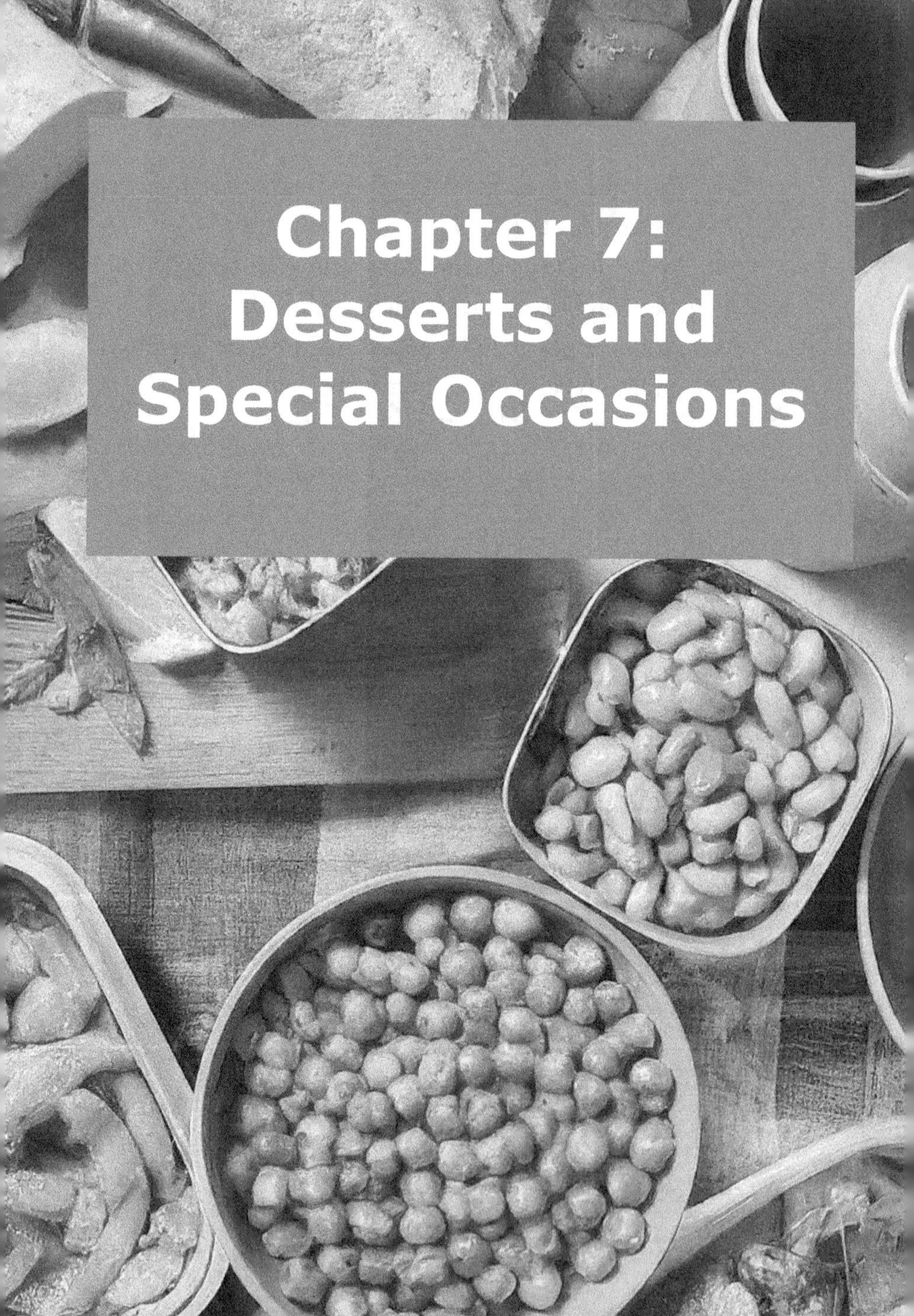

Chapter 7: Desserts and Special Occasions

Diabetic-Friendly Dessert Delights:

Sugar-Free Flourless Chocolate Cookies (Preparation time: 30 minutes):

Ingredients:

- 1/2 cup almond flour
- 1/4 cup unsweetened cocoa powder
- 1/4 cup granulated erythritol (powdered)
- 1/4 cup unsweetened applesauce
- 2 large eggs
- 1/2 teaspoon vanilla extract
- Pinch of salt

Instructions:

1. Preheat oven to 350°F (175°C). Line a baking sheet with parchment paper.
2. In a medium bowl, whisk together almond flour, cocoa powder, and erythritol.
3. In a separate bowl, whisk together applesauce, eggs, vanilla extract, and salt until smooth.
4. Gradually add the wet ingredients to the dry ingredients, mixing until just combined.
5. Drop rounded tablespoons of batter onto the prepared baking sheet, leaving space between each cookie.
6. Bake for 10-12 minutes, or until the edges are slightly firm and the center is set.
7. Let cool on the baking sheet for a few minutes before transferring to a wire rack to cool completely.

Nutritional Information: (per cookie)

- Calories: 120
- Carbohydrates: 4g (net carbs: 2g)
- Fiber: 2g
- Protein: 4g
- Fat: 8g

Tips:

- For a richer flavor, use dark chocolate cocoa powder.
- Add a pinch of espresso powder for extra depth.
- Top the cookies with a sprinkle of flaked sea salt for a sweet and salty contrast.
- Use a cookie scoop for uniform cookies.

Baked Apples with Spiced Quinoa Crumble (Preparation time: 45 minutes):

Ingredients:

- 4 medium apples (e.g., Gala, Fuji)
- 1/2 cup cooked quinoa
- 1/4 cup chopped walnuts or pecans
- 1/2 teaspoon ground cinnamon
- 1/4 teaspoon ground nutmeg
- 1/4 teaspoon ground ginger
- 1 tablespoon maple syrup
- 1/4 cup rolled oats

Instructions:

1. Preheat oven to 375°F (190°C).
2. Wash and core the apples, leaving the bottom intact.
3. In a small bowl, combine cooked quinoa, chopped nuts, cinnamon, nutmeg, ginger, and maple syrup.
4. Fill the apple cavities with the quinoa mixture.
5. Sprinkle the tops of the apples with rolled oats.
6. Place the apples in a baking dish and bake for 25-30 minutes, or until the apples are tender and the crumble is golden brown.

Nutritional Information: (per apple)

- Calories: 250
- Carbohydrates: 40g (net carbs: 30g)
- Fiber: 7g
- Protein: 5g
- Fat: 5g

Tips:

- Use different types of nuts for variety, such as almonds or pistachios.
- Substitute rolled oats with almond flour or coconut flakes for a lower-carb crumble.
- Add a squeeze of lemon juice to the apple filling for a touch of brightness.
- Drizzle the baked apples with a touch of low-fat yogurt or ricotta cheese for an extra protein boost.

Individual Coconut Chia Pudding Parfaits (Preparation time: 15 minutes + overnight chilling):

Ingredients:

- 1 cup unsweetened almond milk
- 1/4 cup chia seeds
- 1/4 cup stevia powder or drops
- 1/2 teaspoon vanilla extract
- 1 cup sliced strawberries
- 1/2 cup blueberries
- 1/4 cup unsweetened shredded coconut

Instructions:

1. In a jar or bowl, whisk together almond milk, chia seeds, stevia, and vanilla extract.
2. Cover the jar or bowl and refrigerate for at least 4 hours, or overnight, until the chia seeds thicken and the pudding develops a gel-like consistency.
3. Layer the chia pudding with sliced strawberries, blueberries, and shredded coconut in individual serving glasses.

Nutritional Information: (per serving)

- Calories: 250
- Carbohydrates: 30g (net carbs: 20g)
- Fiber: 8g
- Protein: 4g
- Fat: 7g

Tips:

- Use different fruits like raspberries, mangoes, or kiwis for variety.
- Add a sprinkle of cocoa powder or chopped dark chocolate for a chocolatey twist.
- Top with a dollop of low-fat yogurt or ricotta cheese for additional protein and creaminess.

No-Bake Mini Cheesecakes with Almond Flour Crust (Preparation time: 30 minutes + chilling):

Ingredients:

Crust:

- 1/2 cup almond flour
- 2 tablespoons melted butter
- Pinch of salt

Filling:

- 8 ounces ricotta cheese
- 4 ounces cream cheese, softened
- 1/4 cup stevia powder or drops
- 1 teaspoon vanilla extract
- 1/4 teaspoon almond extract (optional)
- Fresh berries for topping

Instructions:

1. **Crust:** Combine almond flour, melted butter, and salt in a bowl. Mix well and press into the bottom of individual serving cups or small ramekins. Refrigerate for at least 15 minutes.
2. **Filling:** In a mixing bowl, beat together ricotta cheese, cream cheese, stevia, vanilla extract, and almond extract (if using) until smooth and creamy.

3. Divide the filling evenly among the prepared crusts. Smooth the tops and refrigerate for at least 2 hours, or overnight, until set.

4. Top with fresh berries before serving.

Nutritional Information: (per serving)

- Calories: 250
- Carbohydrates: 10g (net carbs: 5g)
- Fiber: 2g
- Protein: 8g
- Fat: 20g

Tips:

- Use a food processor to easily grind almonds into flour.
- Substitute almond flour with coconut flour for a different flavor and texture.
- Top the cheesecakes with a sprinkle of chopped nuts or seeds for added crunch.
- Dip the berries in a small amount of melted sugar-free chocolate for a decadent touch.

Dark Chocolate Bark with Roasted Nuts and Seeds (Preparation time: 20 minutes):

Ingredients:

- 4 ounces dark chocolate (70% or higher cacao), chopped
- 1/4 cup chopped nuts (e.g., almonds, pecans, pistachios)
- 1/4 cup pumpkin seeds
- 1/4 cup dried cranberries or goji berries

Instructions:

1. Line a baking sheet with parchment paper.
2. Melt the dark chocolate in a microwave-safe bowl on low power, stirring frequently, until smooth.
3. Spread the melted chocolate evenly onto the prepared baking sheet.
4. While the chocolate is still warm, sprinkle with chopped nuts, pumpkin seeds, and dried fruit.
5. Refrigerate for at least 30 minutes, or until the chocolate is set.
6. Break the bark into pieces and enjoy.

Nutritional Information: (per serving)

- Calories: 200
- Carbohydrates: 15g (net carbs: 5g)
- Fiber: 3g
- Protein: 3g
- Fat: 13g

Tips:

- Use different types of nuts and seeds for variety.
- Add a sprinkle of sea salt for a sweet and salty flavor combination.
- Drizzle the bark with a touch of melted sugar-free white chocolate for extra flavor.
- Store the bark in an airtight container in the refrigerator for up to a week.

1. As a registered dietitian with over 20 years of experience, I know how challenging holidays and special occasions can be for managing diabetes. The abundance of tempting treats and rich dishes can easily throw your blood sugar levels off balance. But fear not! With a few mindful adjustments, you can still enjoy festive celebrations without sacrificing your health goals.

2. **Focus on Whole Foods:** This is my golden rule! Instead of processed snacks and sugary desserts, make beautiful and vibrant platters brimming with fresh fruits, roasted vegetables drizzled with herbs and spices, or whole-wheat grain salads packed with protein and fiber. These options offer essential nutrients, fiber for satiety, and keep your blood sugar levels stable.

3. **Portion Control is Key:** Let's be honest, sometimes the sheer variety of holiday spreads can lead to overindulgence. Remember, mindful portions are still enjoyable! Use smaller plates, choose a few items you truly love, and savor each bite. Remember, you can always go back for seconds, but starting smaller helps prevent overdoing it.

4. **Sweeteners with Benefits:** While we're talking mindful enjoyment, let's discuss sweets! Refined sugar can significantly impact blood sugar, so explore natural sweeteners like stevia, erythritol, or monk fruit extract. Remember, even natural sweeteners should be used in moderation.

5. **Potlucks: A Team Effort:** Celebrating with friends and family? Encourage everyone to contribute healthy dishes! This way, you have more control over ingredients and can share a variety of delicious and nutritious options. It's a win-win!

6. **More Than Just Food:** Let's shift the focus sometimes! Plan activities like board games, charades, or even a dance party to keep the emphasis on fun and connection rather than just food. Engaging activities help create lasting memories and manage post-meal blood sugar spikes.

7. **Drink Smart:** Opt for water, unsweetened tea, or sparkling water with a splash of fruit juice for hydration and to avoid sugary drinks that can wreak havoc on your blood sugar. Remember, staying hydrated is key for overall health and digestion.

8. **Mini Treats, Big Satisfaction:** Instead of large, calorie-laden desserts, offer individual portions of healthier indulgences. Think fruit skewers drizzled with a touch of honey, yogurt parfaits with berries and granola, or even sugar-free truffles made with dark chocolate and nut butter. These offer a sweet treat without the sugar overload.

9. **Move It!** After enjoying a delicious meal, get your body moving! Plan a walk around the neighborhood, have a family dance party, or even play some active games. Physical

activity helps digestion, improves blood sugar control, and prevents that feeling of being overly full.

10. **Quality over Quantity:** This extends beyond just sweets! Choose smaller portions of high-quality ingredients that offer more nutritional value. Opt for dark chocolate with a higher cocoa percentage instead of milk chocolate, or savor fresh berries rich in antioxidants and fiber instead of processed treats.

11. **Celebrate Your Way:** Remember, holidays are about creating memories and strengthening bonds with loved ones. Don't let food stress overshadow the joy of celebration. Focus on laughter, connection, and the spirit of the season, and enjoy mindful, delicious treats along the way!

By implementing these tips and consulting with your healthcare team, you can have a joyful and healthy holiday season that celebrates you and your well-being!

BONUS CHAPTER

DIABETES MEAL PLAN TRACKER

DIABETES MEAL PLAN

Tracker

1200-CALORIE LOW-CARB DIET PLAN

	protein	carbs	fat	total calories
meals	15% -30%	**40% - 65%**	20%-35%	1200 to 1500 calories

DAILY CALORIES SAMPLE

	protein	**carbs**	**fat**	**total calories**
Mushroom & lentil scramble	20 gm	25 gm	15 gm	350 calories
Tuscan white bean soup with kale & sausage	25 gm	45gm	20 gm	400 calories
Salmon and veggie stir-fry with Quinoa	35 gm	30 gm	20 gm	400 calories
Roasted beet chips	1 gm	8 gm	2 gm	52 calories
total	81 gm	78 gm	57 gm	1202 kcal

DIABETES DIET MONTHLY TRACKER

DIABETES DIET MONTHLY TRACKER | MONTH _____________

date	meal	drink	protein	carbs	fat	cal.
1						
2						
3						
4						
5						
6						
7						
8						
9						
10						
11						
12						
13						
14						
15						
16						
17						
18						
19						
20						
21						
22						
23						
24						
25						
266						
27						
28						
29						
30						
31						

DIABETES DIET MONTHLY TRACKER | MONTH _________

date	meal	drink	protein	carbs	fat	cal.
1						
2						
3						
4						
5						
6						
7						
8						
9						
10						
11						
12						
13						
14						
15						
16						
17						
18						
19						
20						
21						
22						
23						
24						
25						
266						
27						
28						
29						
30						
31						

DIABETES DIET MONTHLY TRACKER | MONTH __________

date	meal	drink	protein	carbs	fat	cal.
1						
2						
3						
4						
5						
6						
7						
8						
9						
10						
11						
12						
13						
14						
15						
16						
17						
18						
19						
20						
21						
22						
23						
24						
25						
266						
27						
28						
29						
30						
31						

DIABETES DIET MONTHLY TRACKER | MONTH __________

date	meal	drink	protein	carbs	fat	cal.
1						
2						
3						
4						
5						
6						
7						
8						
9						
10						
11						
12						
13						
14						
15						
16						
17						
18						
19						
20						
21						
22						
23						
24						
25						
266						
27						
28						
29						
30						
31						

DIABETES DIET MONTHLY TRACKER | MONTH __________

date	meal	drink	protein	carbs	fat	cal.
1						
2						
3						
4						
5						
6						
7						
8						
9						
10						
11						
12						
13						
14						
15						
16						
17						
18						
19						
20						
21						
22						
23						
24						
25						
266						
27						
28						
29						
30						
31						

DIABETES DIET MONTHLY TRACKER | MONTH ___________

date	meal	drink	protein	carbs	fat	cal.
1						
2						
3						
4						
5						
6						
7						
8						
9						
10						
11						
12						
13						
14						
15						
16						
17						
18						
19						
20						
21						
22						
23						
24						
25						
266						
27						
28						
29						
30						
31						

DIABETES DIET MONTHLY TRACKER | MONTH __________

date	meal	drink	protein	carbs	fat	cal.
1						
2						
3						
4						
5						
6						
7						
8						
9						
10						
11						
12						
13						
14						
15						
16						
17						
18						
19						
20						
21						
22						
23						
24						
25						
266						
27						
28						
29						
30						
31						

DIABETES DIET MONTHLY TRACKER | MONTH _________

date	meal	drink	protein	carbs	fat	cal.
1						
2						
3						
4						
5						
6						
7						
8						
9						
10						
11						
12						
13						
14						
15						
16						
17						
18						
19						
20						
21						
22						
23						
24						
25						
266						
27						
28						
29						
30						
31						

DIABETES DIET MONTHLY TRACKER | MONTH __________

date	meal	drink	protein	carbs	fat	cal.
1						
2						
3						
4						
5						
6						
7						
8						
9						
10						
11						
12						
13						
14						
15						
16						
17						
18						
19						
20						
21						
22						
23						
24						
25						
266						
27						
28						
29						
30						
31						

DIABETES DIET MONTHLY TRACKER | MONTH ___________

date	meal	drink	protein	carbs	fat	cal.
1						
2						
3						
4						
5						
6						
7						
8						
9						
10						
11						
12						
13						
14						
15						
16						
17						
18						
19						
20						
21						
22						
23						
24						
25						
266						
27						
28						
29						
30						
31						

DIABETES DIET MONTHLY TRACKER | MONTH _______________

date	meal	drink	protein	carbs	fat	cal.
1						
2						
3						
4						
5						
6						
7						
8						
9						
10						
11						
12						
13						
14						
15						
16						
17						
18						
19						
20						
21						
22						
23						
24						
25						
266						
27						
28						
29						
30						
31						

DIABETES DIET MONTHLY TRACKER | MONTH _______

date	meal	drink	protein	carbs	fat	cal.
1						
2						
3						
4						
5						
6						
7						
8						
9						
10						
11						
12						
13						
14						
15						
16						
17						
18						
19						
20						
21						
22						
23						
24						
25						
266						
27						
28						
29						
30						
31